the

POSITIVELY
AWESOME

JOURNAL

First published in the United Kingdom in 2021 by
Pavilion
An imprint of HarperCollins*Publishers*
1 London Bridge Street
London SE1 9GF

www.harpercollins.co.uk

HarperCollins*Publishers*
Macken House
39/40 Mayor Street Upper
Dublin 1
DO1 C9W8
Ireland

ISBN 9781911663010

A CIP catalogue record for this book is available from the
British Library.

10 9 8 7 6 5 4 3 2

Reproduction by Rival Colour Ltd, UK
Printed and bound in China by RR Donnelley APS

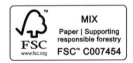

This book is produced from independently certified FSC™ paper
to ensure responsible forest management.

For more information visit: www.harpercollins.co.uk/green

the
POSITIVELY AWESOME

JOURNAL

STACIE SWIFT

PAVILION

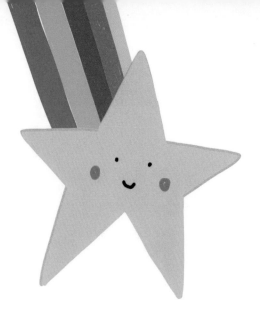

For my wonderful Grandad Ken.

And my legendary Nanny Mary.

xxx

This book belongs to:

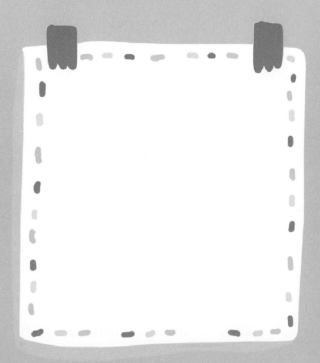

HELLO

This journal is a space to record the good and bad days.

To work through the ups and downs.

And a place to focus on self-care and positive well-being.

It's for you to use
whenever and wherever.

To fill in, to share,
to encourage.

It's yours.

A reminder that you
matter, too.

ME

Fill in this space with a self-portrait.

Don't want to draw yourself?
Draw a series of objects or colours
that best represent you!

Write 5 positive statements about yourself.

_____

_____

_____

_____

_____

Come back to this page if ever you need
a reminder of who you really are.

Self-Care
Tool Kit

What are the things that help you
to best look after yourself - both
your mental and physical wellness?

Create a tool kit that you can
refer to when you need to restore
some balance.
A collection of resources and
activities that will help you
to feel brighter.

You don't have to do them all at
once, take each day as it comes.

_____

Some ideas of what to include:

* journalling * nature * cooking *
* taking medication * cleaning *
* therapy * crafting * hot baths *

Create a drawing / list / collage of your kit.

PLAN YOUR IDEAL DAY

Our days very rarely go exactly to plan -
they are filled with countless
challenges, obstacles and distractions.

Write down what your perfect day
would look like.

We can't stop the imperfections from
happening, but we can prioritize, form
new habits and acknowledge the things
that matter most and make us happiest.

Which aspects of your ideal day can
you safeguard or implement into your
normal routine?

(If things don't work out today, there's always tomorrow.)

Morning

Afternoon

Evening

Night

IT's okay TO PUT
YOURSELF FIRST.

MY WEEKLY FEELINGS FORECAST

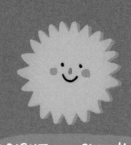

BRIGHT + SUNNY

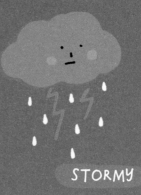

STORMY

monday

tuesday

wednesday

thursday

friday

saturday

sunday

Tick a box each day to keep a
record of your feelings this week.

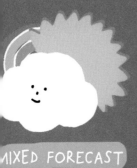

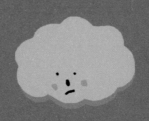

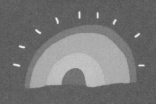

MIXED FORECAST

CLOUDY

BRILLIANT

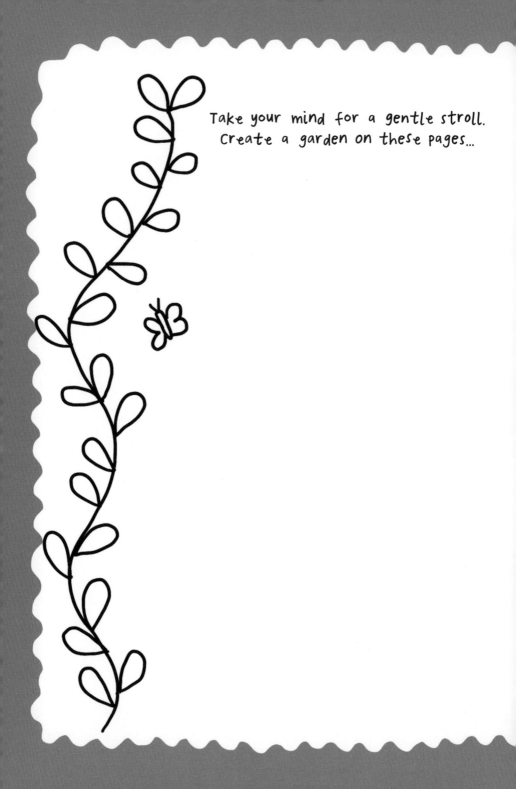

Take your mind for a gentle stroll.
Create a garden on these pages...

THE NOT-TO-DO LIST

Our to-do lists are never-ending but we rarely stop to focus on the things we should take a step back from.

The not-to-dos.

Write your list of don'ts.

Some ideas:

* Don't compare myself to others

* Stop looking at my phone before bed

* Don't avoid making important decisions

* Don't decline offers of help

Draw your
favourite outfit.

Something that
makes you feel
your best,
twinkliest self.

Give yourself
permission to
wear it whenever
you need a boost.
Not just for a
special occasion;
you deserve nice
things in the
here and now, too.

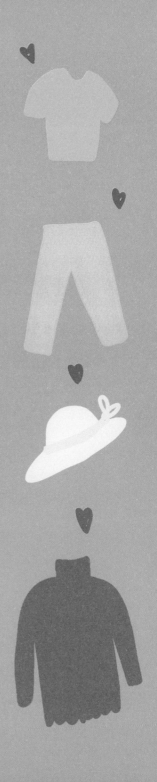

FOR WHEN YOU FEEL WORRIED

Use these pages to track your feelings
and work through your worries.

What's worrying me?

What negative thoughts am I having?

What are some balanced thoughts
or positive potential outcomes?

* it'll be okay

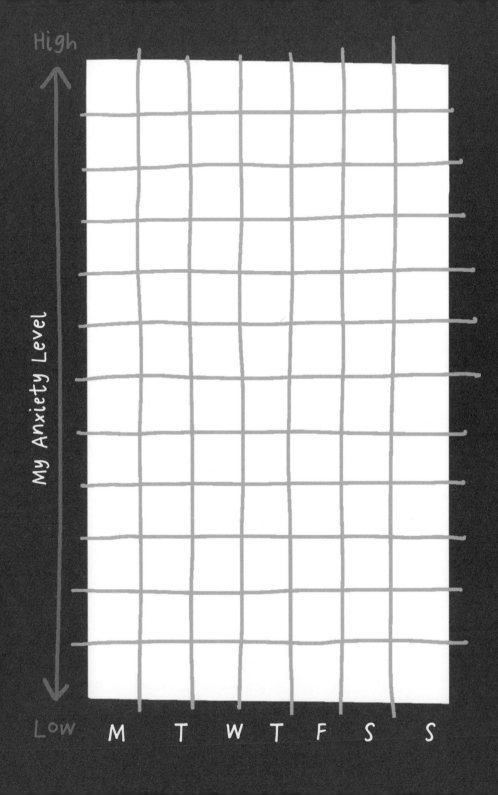

High

My Anxiety Level

Low   M   M   T   W   T   F   S   S

It's okay...

to do less

to prioritize
self-care

to give yourself
room to grow

to expect more

to be learning

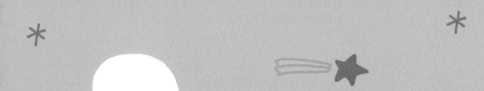

PEOPLE WHO

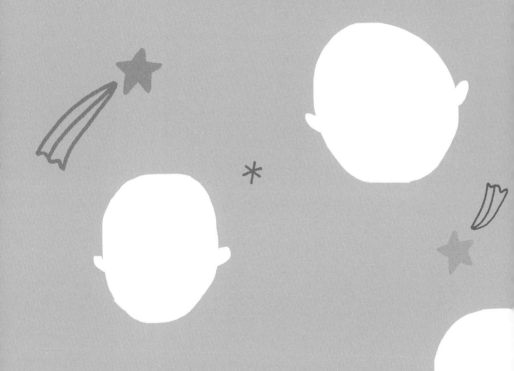

Your best mates, a friendly barista,
the stranger who says good morning
on your commute... doodle in the people
who add some sparkle to your everyday.

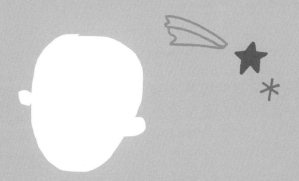

MAKE LIFE SPARKLIER

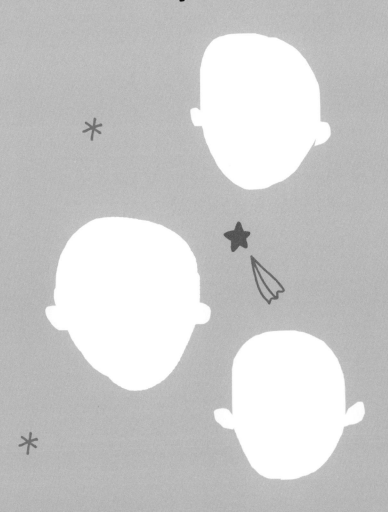

Reflect back on your feelings forecast from a few pages ago. Now you've had a bit of time to review, what made the sunny days brighter?

Focus on these positives.

Try to add some more
sunshine into this week.

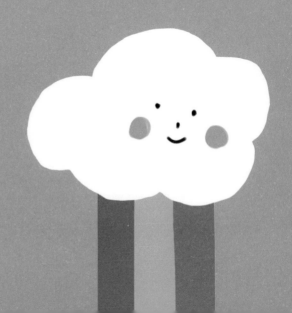

NOTES

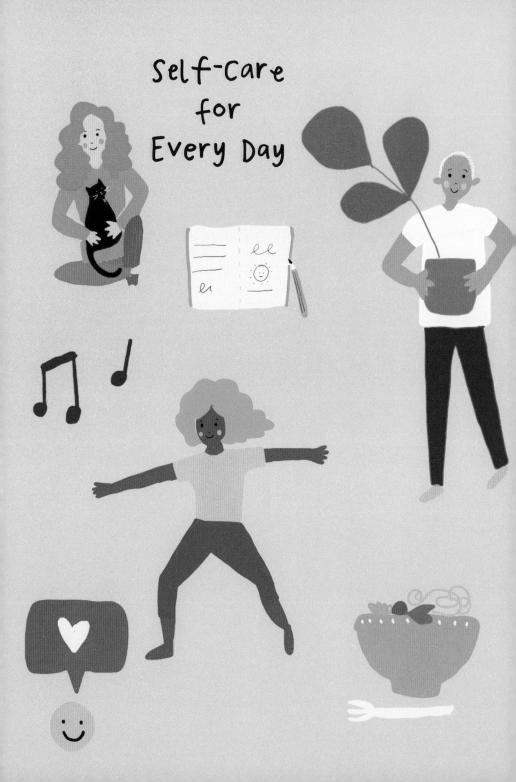

* Make a large cup of your favourite hot drink. Have a mindful few moments to enjoy it without distraction

* Embrace nature, step outside or add some greenery to your home

* Tidy and organize your space

* Move your body - dance, do yoga, stretch in your chair

* Enjoy positive posts online

* Get to bed early

* Find a cute animal to cuddle

* Prepare a nutritious meal

* Read a good book

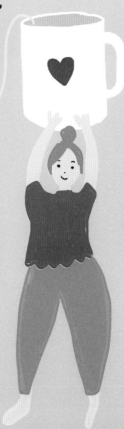

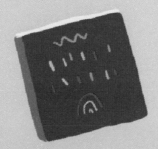

Reminder:

Treat yourself with the same

care and kindness you show to

those you love most.

Look after yourself.

Plan a ten-minute task or
activity that is just for you.
Do it today.

Self-care isn't selfish.

WINNER WINNER EASY DINNER

It's tiring making decisions, especially when
we aren't feeling our best.

Plan ahead for the days you have decision fatigue -
fill these plates with quick, nourishing meals to make
next time you're struggling to decide on dinner.

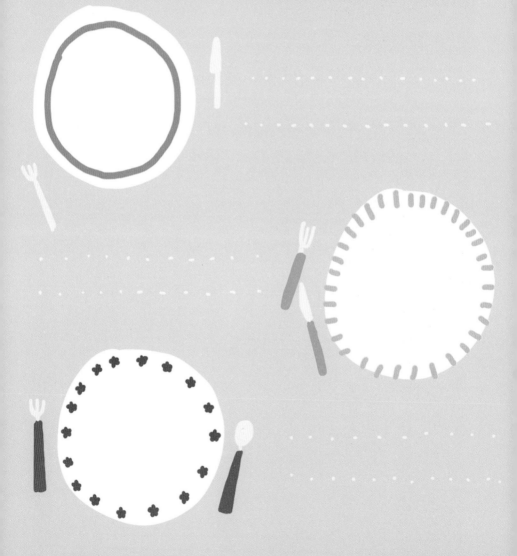

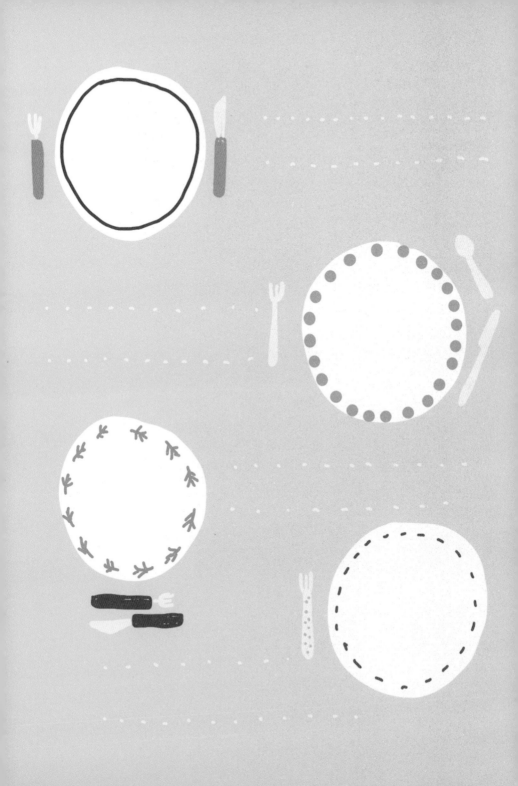

EVERYDAY WINS

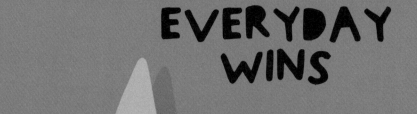

Each day is made up of lots of small victories - what are yours?

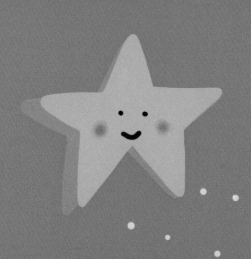

The little things add up.

ENOUGH

You are enough.
Even when you don't feel it.
When self-doubt sneaks in and your
mind is full of perceived shortcomings
and imperfections.

On the days you feel like you should have
done more (had more patience, pushed a bit harder,
ticked more off the to-do list) remember:

You are doing your best.
You are doing what you can, with
what you have, each day.

IS ENOUGH

I am a good enough...

I am good enough at...

I'm not perfect, but I'm...

I am good enough and did my best...

I am good enough even when...

Draw a map of your favourite place to rest and restore. You may not be able to be there physically right now, but revisit it in your mind. Focus on the feeling of calm and contentment it brings.

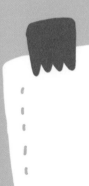

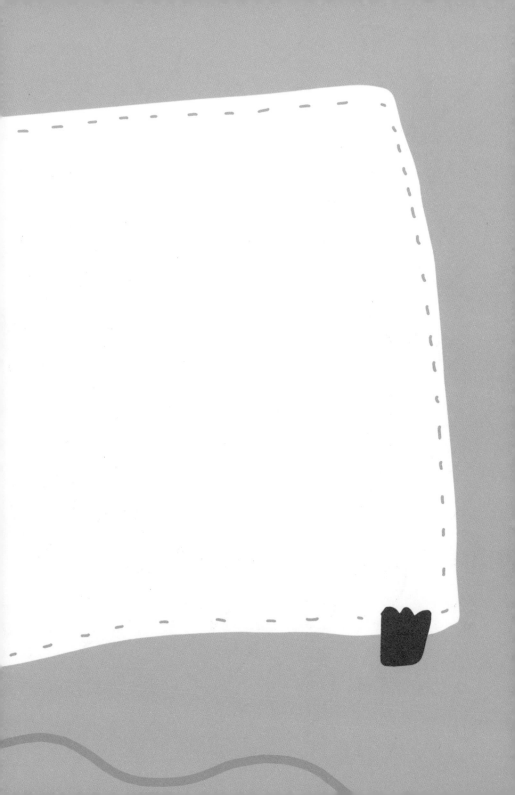

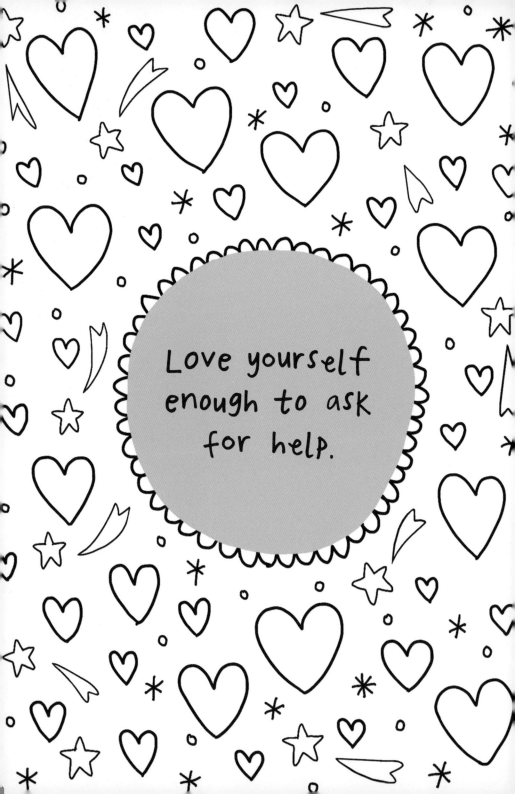

Love yourself enough to ask for help.

People and places I can turn to...

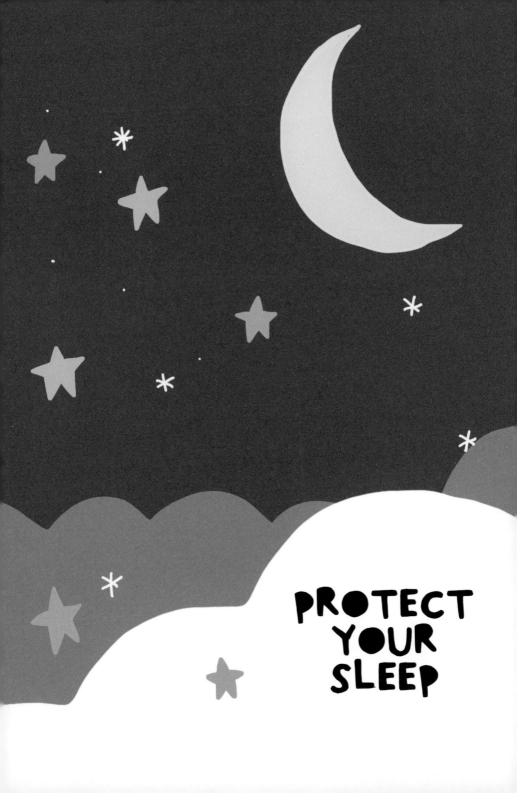

PROTECT
YOUR
SLEEP

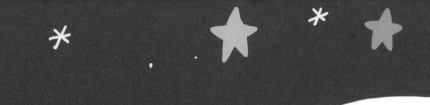

Avoid too much caffeine

Create a worry list to try
to quell those 3am anxieties

Read a book before bed

Leave your phone in another
room and reduce screen time
at night

Make your room as dark
and cosy as you can

Try to stick to a
sleep routine

DREAM LOG

What do you dream about?

Add a new self-care habit into your routine - meditate, drink more water, enforce your boundaries...

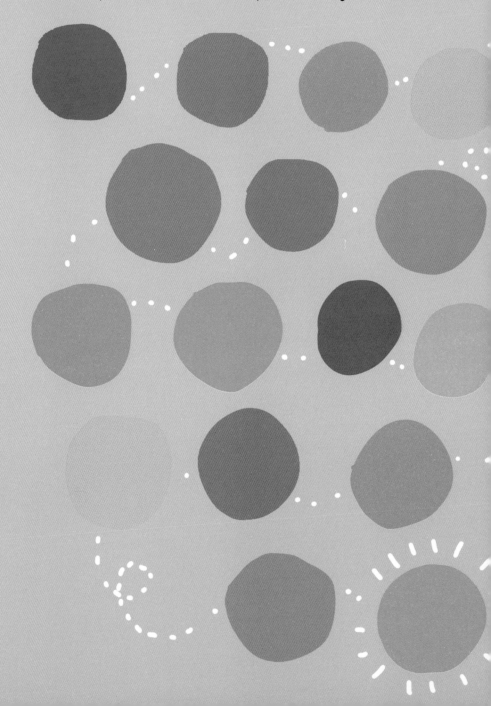

Aim to complete your new act of self-care each
day for 30 days - track your daily progress by
marking a circle on the chart.

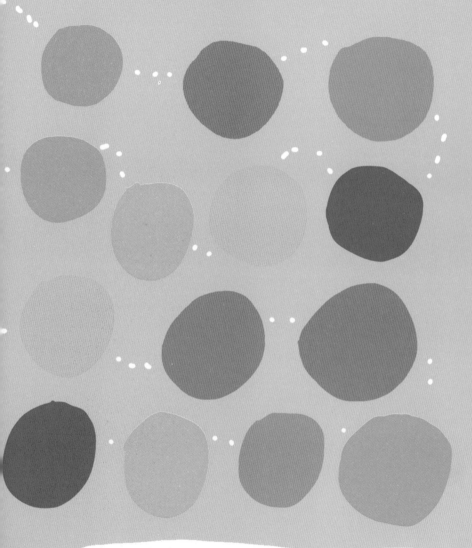

MY NEW SELF-CARE HABIT IS

DO YOU NEED A PICK-ME-UP?

YES!

ARE YOU UP TO LEAVING THE HOUSE?

I AM

DO YOU WANT COMPANY?

NO

YES!

MEET A FRIEND FOR CAKE

GO FOR A STROLL AND SMILE AT ALL OF THE DOGS YOU SEE

NOT TODAY

HOW MUCH ENERGY DO YOU HAVE?

A LITTLE

A LOT

NONE

TIDY AND ORGANIZE YOUR SPACE

REST WITH A SNACK AND A BOOK

PUT YOUR FAVOURITE SONG ON AND HAVE A DANCE

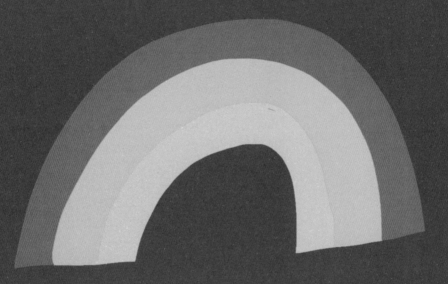

Let yourself focus.

What are your biggest distractions?
How can you juggle less and focus more?

Consider blocking apps, turning off notifications, working
away from the TV, implementing new routines...

Stick a photo here of a past you -
you as a child, or when you most
needed some love and kindness.

Write this version of you a
letter, tell them all the things
you wanted or needed to hear.

♥ XOXO

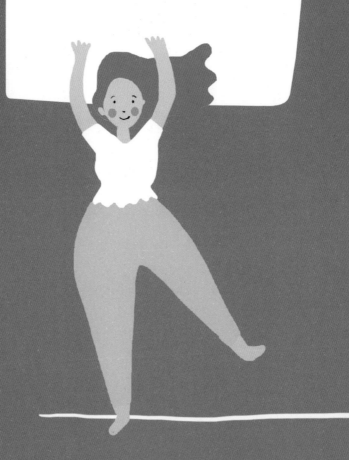

Now tell
yourself,
too.

READING LOG

Date	Title	Comments

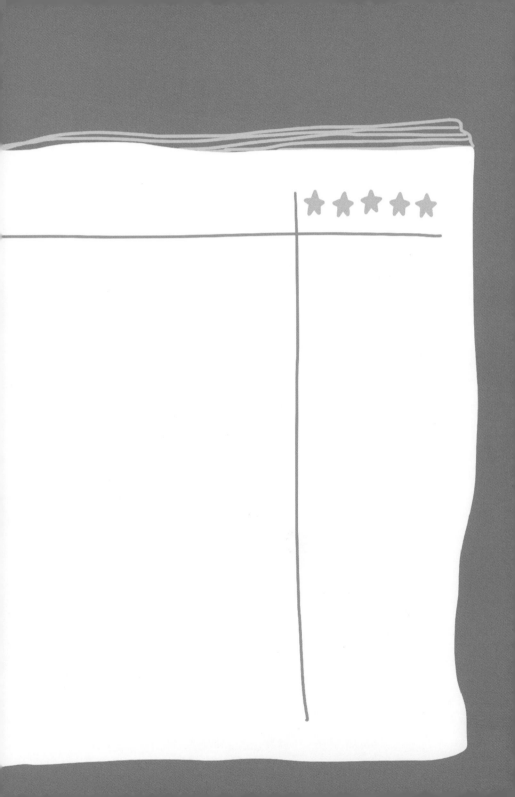

GO OUTSIDE

Get out into nature, take a mindful walk.

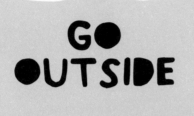

Take notice of how many
dogs you see.

Listen out for birds.

Enjoy the feeling of
the breeze, or rain, or
sun on your face.

Walk a route you don't
usually take, try to keep
your mind only on
the present.

One foot in front of
the other.

THOUGHTS aren't FACTS.

Use this space to brain dump your thoughts.

A SOUNDTRACK FOR SUNNY DAYS

SONGS FOR STORMY DAYS

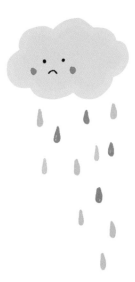

A WEEK OF GRATITUDE

Even on our hardest days we have things to be thankful for.
There may be times when we need to look a little harder to see the good...

... but there is always a positive to be found.

Practising gratitude can help us feel brighter and uplifts us during the difficult times.
It has been proven to benefit both our mental and physical health.

Commit to recording one thing you are thankful for each day, big or small.

Monday

_____

Tuesday

_____

Wednesday

_____

Thursday

_____

Friday

_____

Saturday

_____

Sunday

_____

Keep shining.

Spreading
kindness

Time to
rest

Reading
good books

Good
things to
prioritize

Family

Mental and
physical health

Good
friends

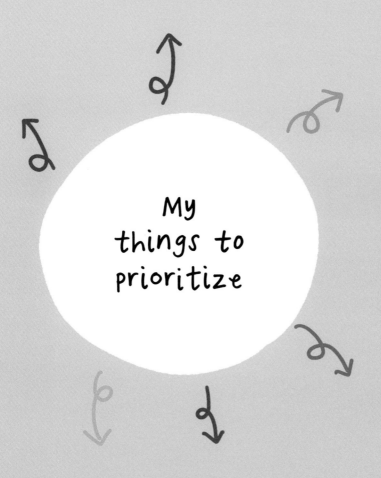

My
things to
prioritize

NOTES

YOU MIGHT NOT ALWAYS FEEL IT,

BUT YOU'RE SO VERY BRAVE and

SO MUCH STRONGER THAN

YOU REALIZE.

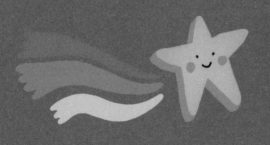

YOU ARE STRONG

EVEN WHEN YOU NEED HELP
EVEN WHEN LIFE FEELS HEAVY
EVEN WHEN YOU STRUGGLE
EVEN WHEN YOU STOP AND TRY AGAIN

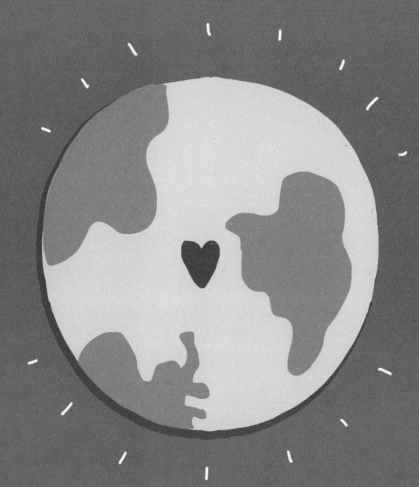

SMALL ACTS CAN
CHANGE THE WORLD

I PLEDGE TO ...

♥ . . . .

♥ . . . .

♥ . . . .

Choose three small, achievable
actions that will make the planet
happier or the world a bit brighter.
All of the little things add up.

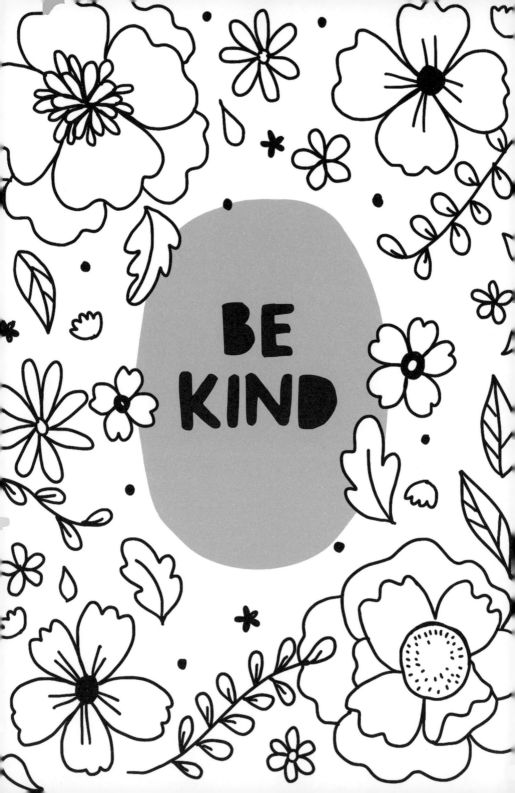

Kindness isn't just for giving to other people. How can you practise being kinder to yourself?

Stop.

breathe in through your
nose for 4 seconds.

hold that deep breath
for 7 seconds.

exhale through your
mouth for 8 seconds.

Circle of Self-acceptance

What flaws can you embrace? Colour and label this circle, use these pages to recognize what makes you unique (and human).

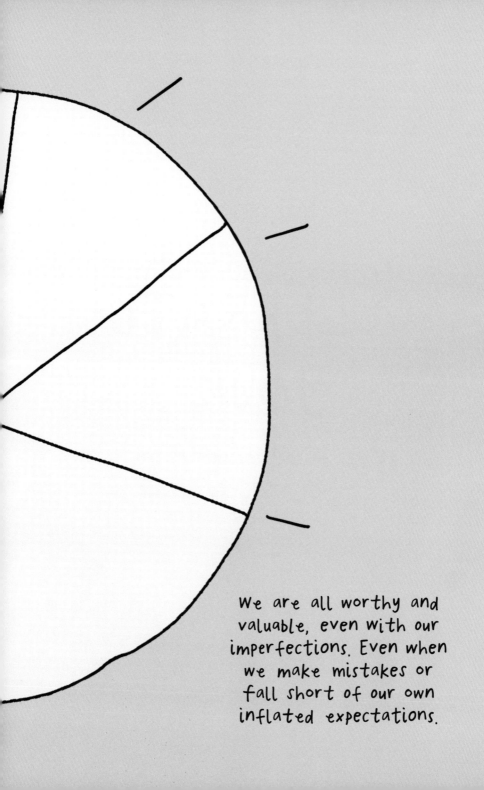

We are all worthy and valuable, even with our imperfections. Even when we make mistakes or fall short of our own inflated expectations.

CELEBRATE YOUR PROGRESS.

We might not be where we want to be, but
every step in the right direction matters.
Start a list of progress to celebrate.

Not perfect, but better.

We do not always feel courageous, and yet each and every day we are facing our fears: digging deep, demonstrating our strength and resilience in spite of ourselves.

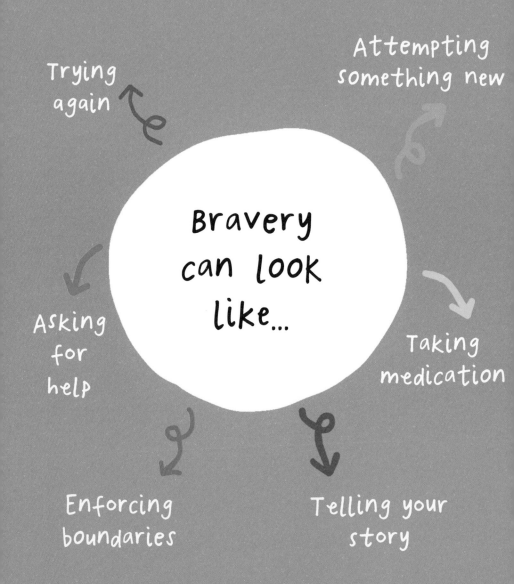

Trying again

Attempting something new

Bravery can look like...

Asking for help

Taking medication

Enforcing boundaries

Telling your story

Give yourself credit for all of the things you do, the obstacles you overcome, the small battles you win, day after day.

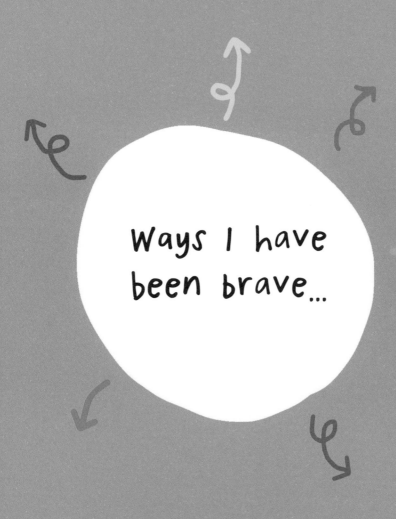

Ways I have been brave...

What are you carrying
that's heavy?

Put it in this box,
I'll hold it for a while.

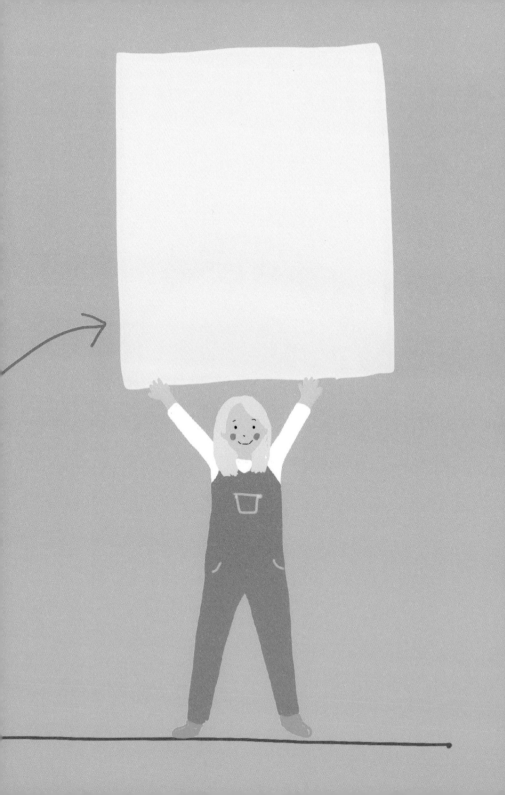

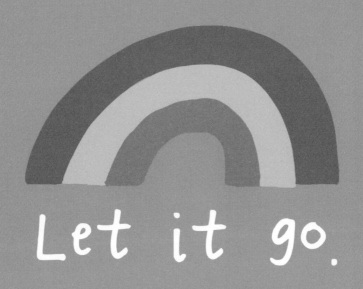

Let it go.

Things to let go of:

Past mistakes

Other people's opinions

The weight of expectation

Shame

Comparing yourself to others

Try something new.

Write a poem
or a haiku.

It doesn't have
to be good.

It's okay just to do
things for fun!

GLAD YOU WERE HERE

Write a postcard to someone who has impacted your life for the better.

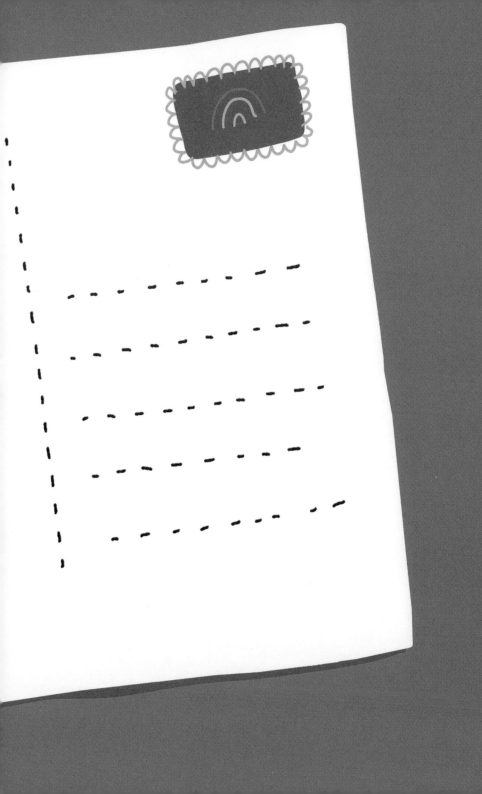

MINE

What are the things that
make your heart feel fullest?

OTHERS

What are the things that you
can do to show appreciation for
others? Keep filling up hearts.

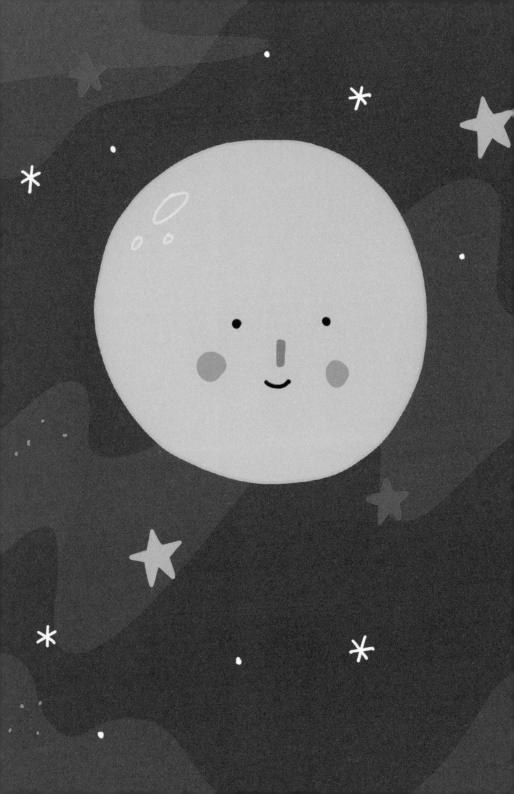

SOME SPACE

GIVE YOURSELF
the CREDIT
YOU DESERVE.

A list of things I've achieved despite my fears and anxieties...

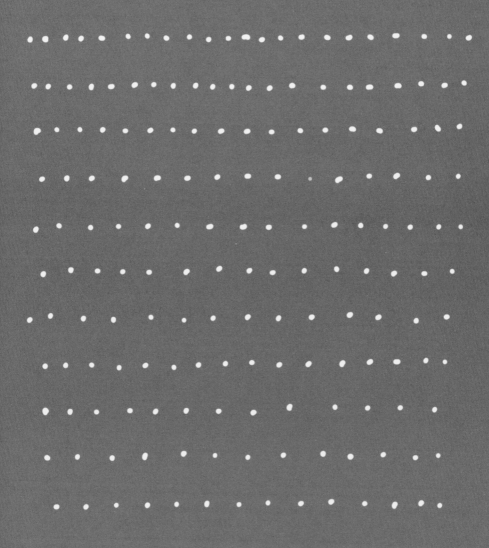

It's okay to cry.

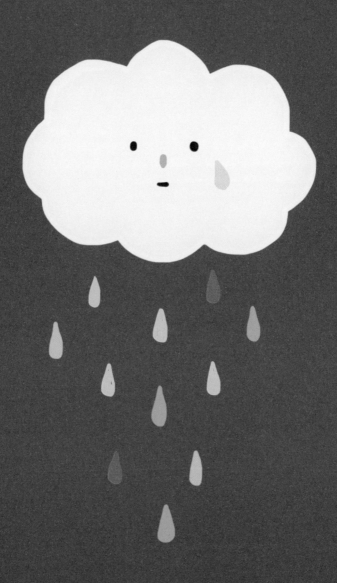

Reasons I've cried:

Crying is good for our mental health:
it releases stress; produces more
feel-good chemicals; helps us to self-soothe
and can help us connect with others.

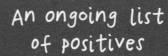

An ongoing list
of positives

- _____
- _____
- _____
- _____
- _____
- _____
- _____
- _____
- _____

Record happy thoughts, compliments, good news... LOOK here when you need a smile.

KEEP GROWING

Nurture the ways in which you'd like to grow, the qualities and attributes you'd like to see bloom.

What are they?

Label the pots with ideas for self-improvement.

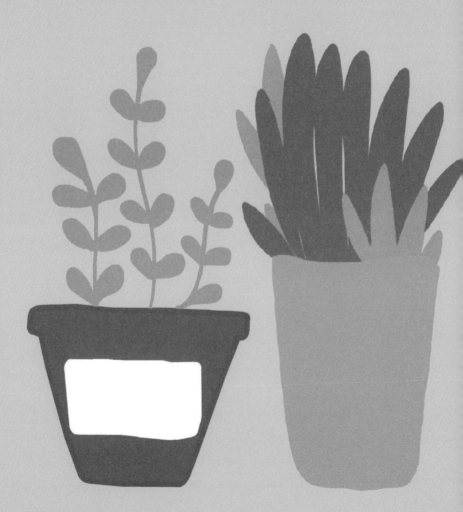

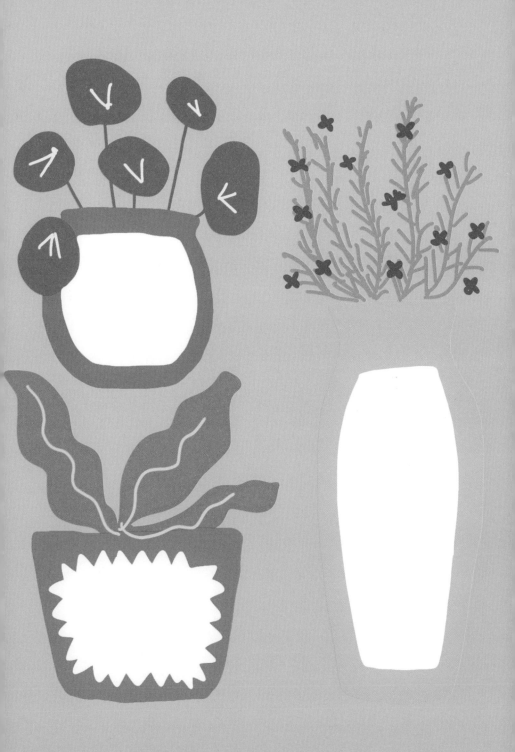

LOOK HOW FAR YOU'VE COME

We get so caught up in what's happening next - spending our time looking forward and chasing bigger goals.

It's easy to miss all the progress we've made to get this far. We don't stop to appreciate the effort we've put in to get here.

Take some time to reflect on your accomplishments. You've achieved so, so much.

progress in the last 6 months:

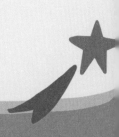

progress in the last year:

progress in the last 5 years:

It's okay to keep growing and changing.

You don't have to make yourself small or compromise your personal journey to keep other people happy.

GROWTH CAN BE

Messy

Slow

Uncomfortable

Challenging

Relationship-changing

Feeling like an imposter?

It's okay, you aren't alone in having these thoughts...

Speak to a friend for some support (and cheerleading).

Take a minute to write down all of your qualifications or skills.

Now note down all of your lived experiences.

Go ahead and say something
nice to yourself...
e.g. 'I am good enough.
I deserve success'.

Feel any better?
(If not, repeat the previous steps.)

Remember:
You have value.
You are ACCOMPLISHED.
You are worthy.

YOU ARE ENOUGH

PASSING
THOUGHTS

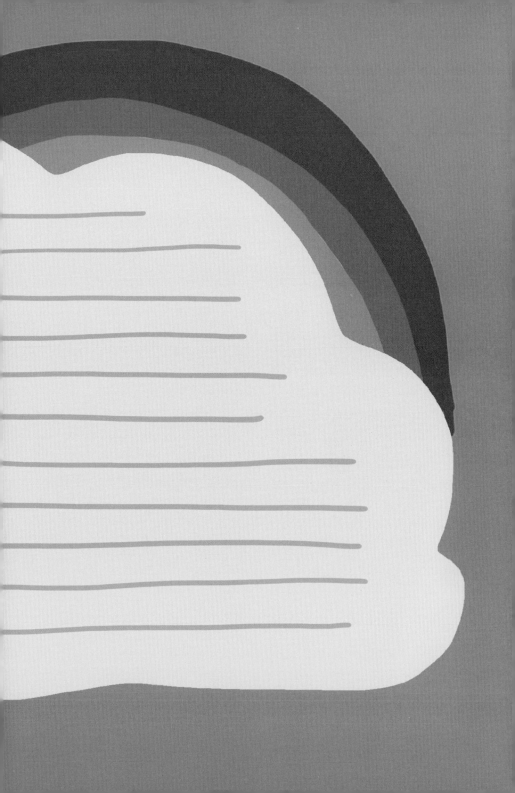

YOU BELONG HERE

If you feel out of place, undeserving or like you aren't good enough, fill in these pages.

When do I feel like I don't belong?

What is my biggest concern? How likely is this to happen?

I am not a fraud; I am good enough;
it's okay to be out of my comfort zone;
I am not an imposter.

TEN REASONS I BELONG HERE:

1

2

3

4

5

6

7

8

9

10

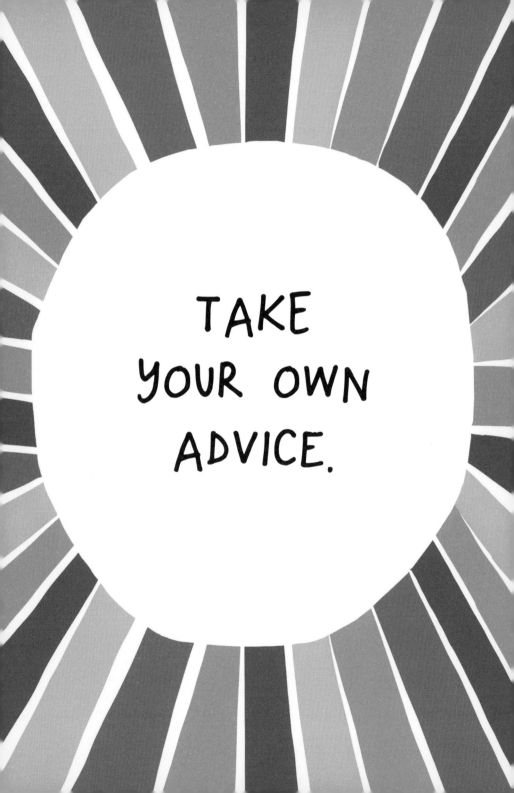

It's much easier to give advice to others than to practise self-compassion and act upon our own words of wisdom.

Treat yourself like a friend,
what piece of advice should you listen to?

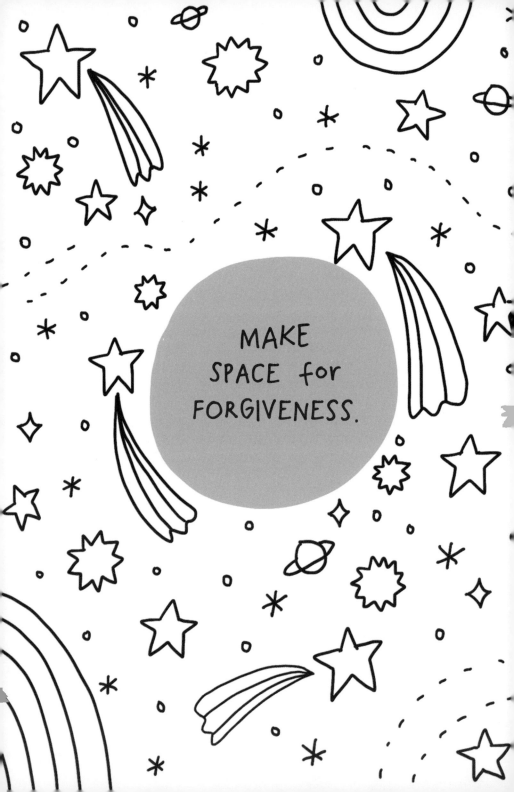

MAKE
SPACE for
FORGIVENESS.

Things I forgive myself for:

Things I'd like to be forgiven for:

People I have forgiven:

Don't hide your magic,
don't stop shining.

Other people may not appreciate
or understand the way you sparkle.
Don't dull your shine to please
anyone else or to fit a mould.
Keep being the brightest, truest
version of you.

You're allowed to be exactly
who you are.

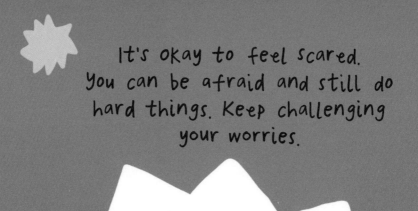

It's okay to feel scared.
You can be afraid and still do
hard things. Keep challenging
your worries.

Something I was anxious about...

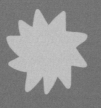

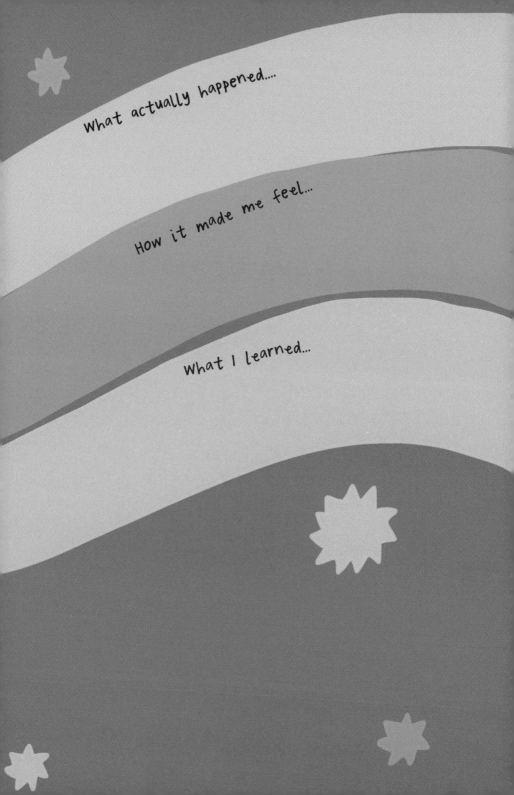

What actually happened....

How it made me feel...

What I learned...

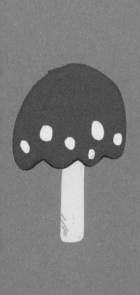
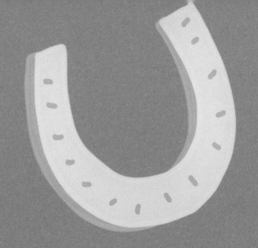

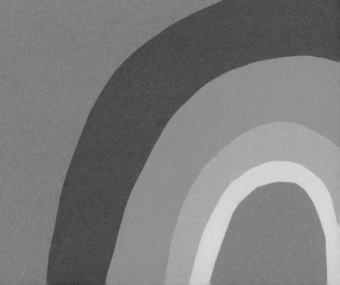

MAKE
YOUR
OWN
LUCK

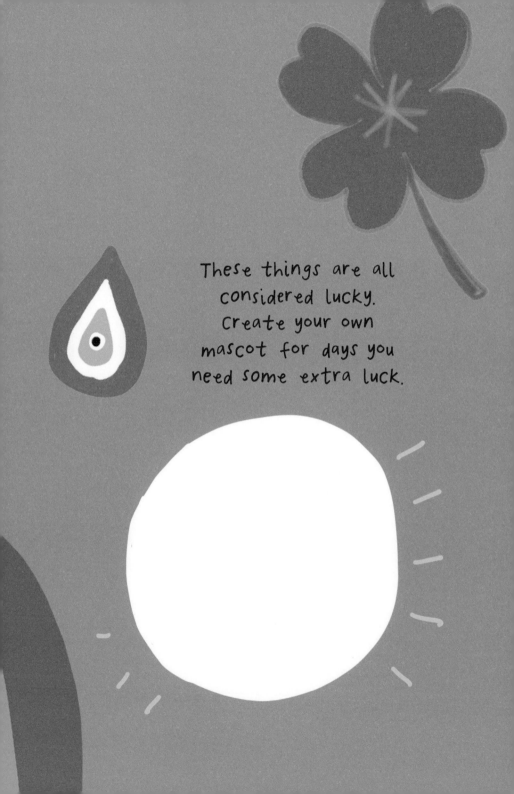

These things are all
considered lucky.
Create your own
mascot for days you
need some extra luck.

Keep pushing through the darkness,
face towards the sun,

Keep growing, slow and steady,
Petals blooming one by one.

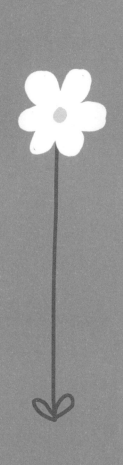

Fill these
pages with
happy memories.

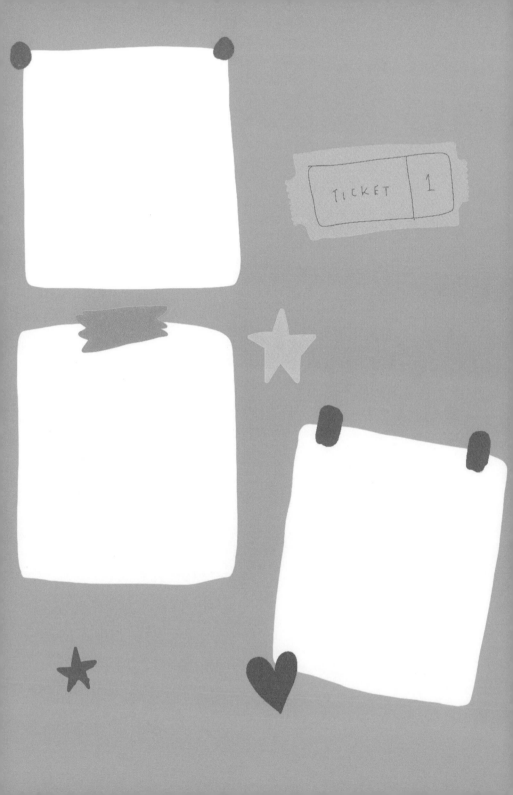

TICKET 1

SLOWLY BUT SURELY

Set yourself a challenge.
Break it down into 8 steps.
Write each one next to a flower.

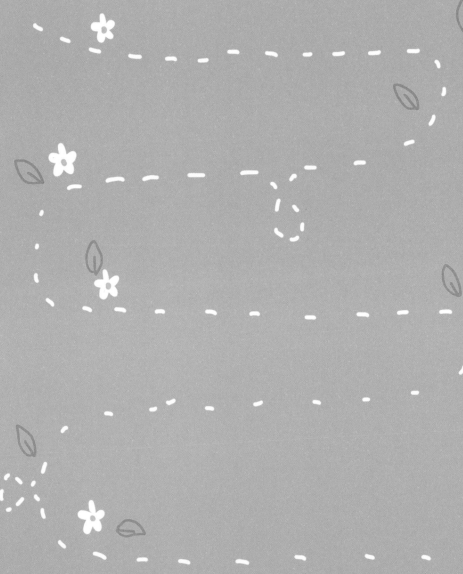

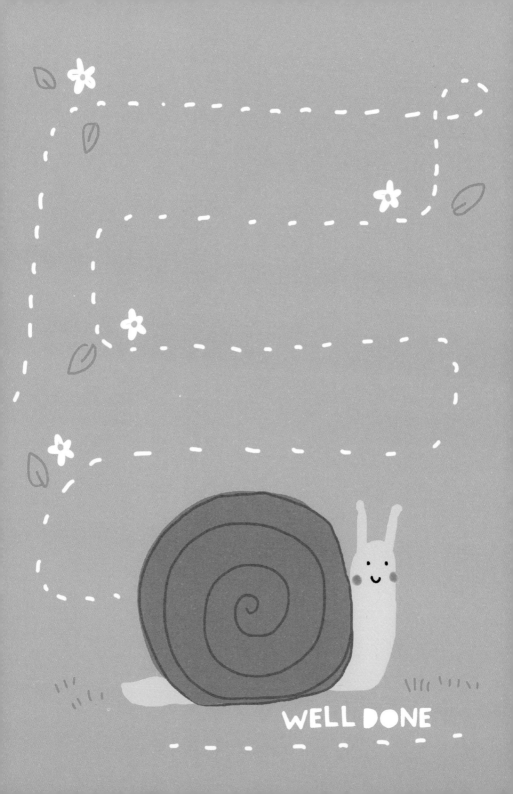

WELL DONE

A safe space to say all of the things that are difficult to speak out loud.

Draw yourself shouting onto the pages. Don't hold back.

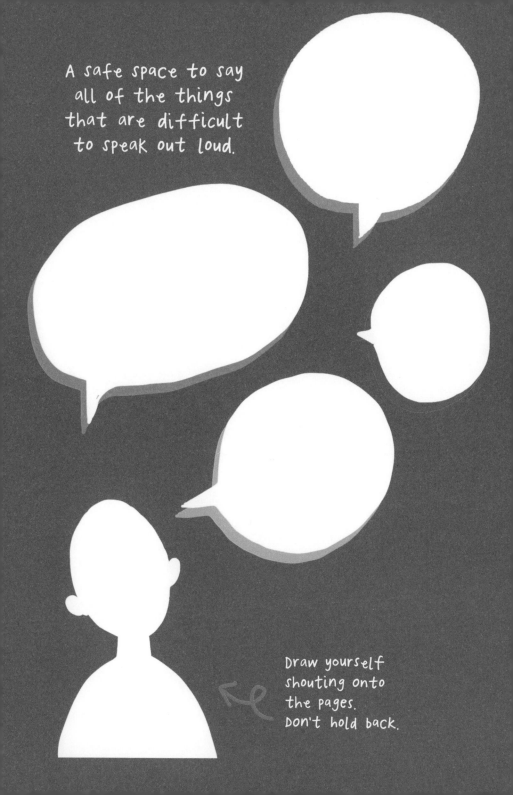

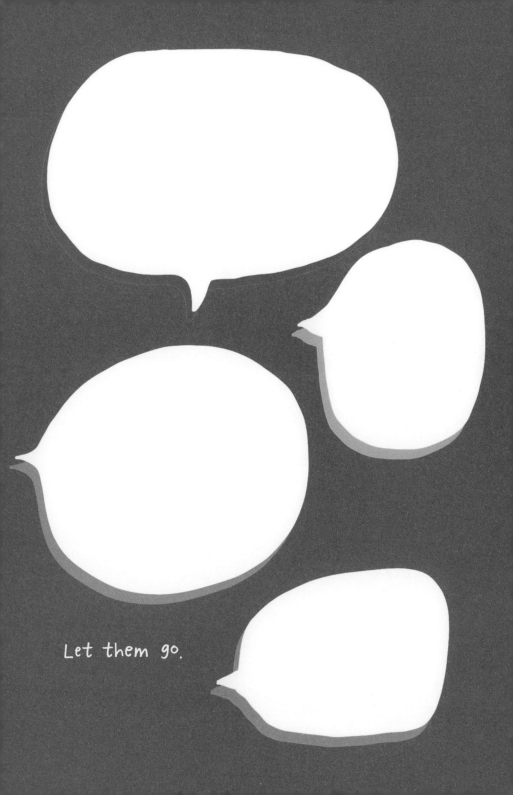

Let them go.

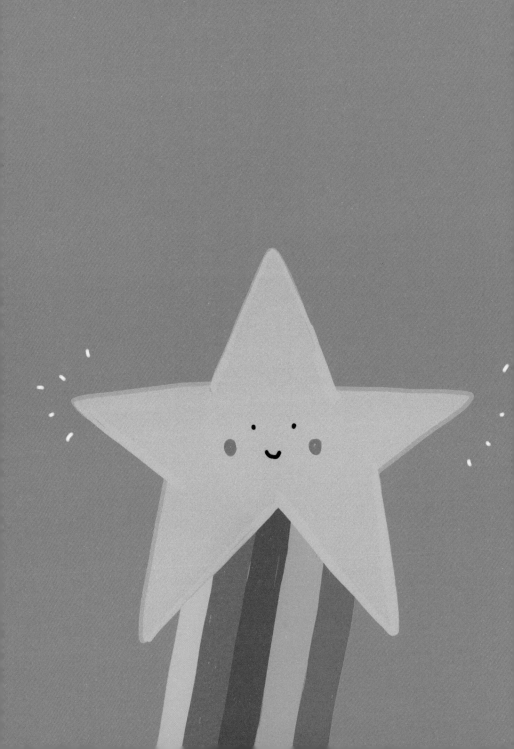

Adulting is hard. There's not nearly enough reward for all of the difficult, wobbly bits. Give yourself a gold star every time you do something that deserves praise. Fill the pages - embrace your inner child.

What are the things that
weigh you down?

The secrets we carry, the shame
we cannot shake, we all have the
waves of these burdens crash
over us and make us feel out
of our depth.

Write them in the bottle.
When it's full, scribble them out.
Let those feelings wash away.

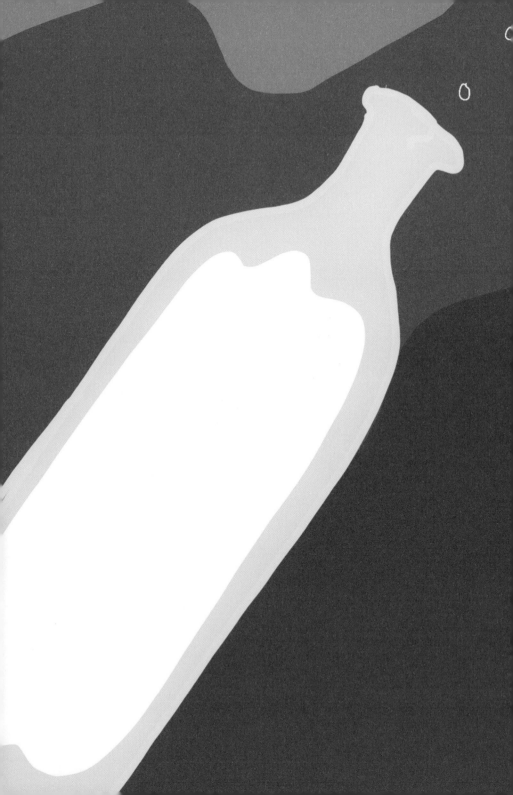

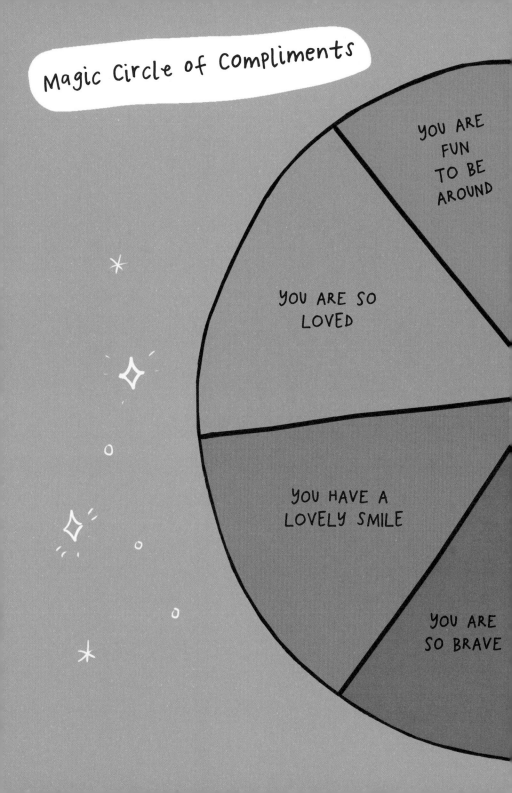

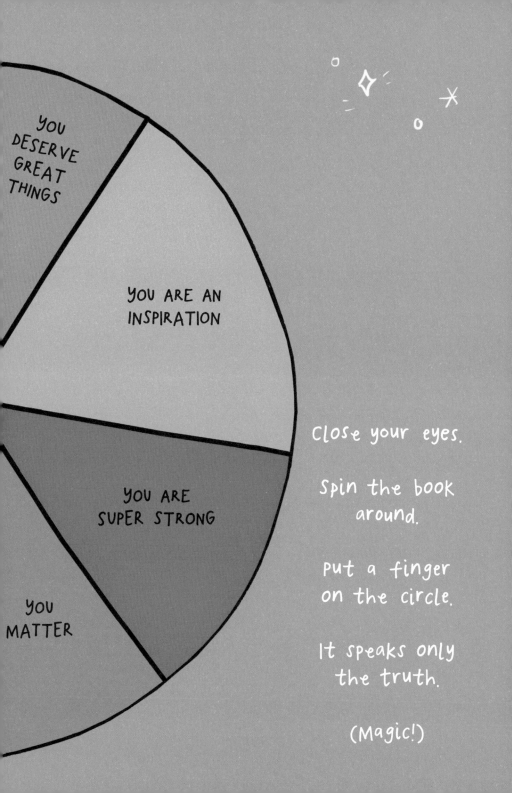

YOU
DESERVE
GREAT
THINGS

YOU ARE AN
INSPIRATION

YOU ARE
SUPER STRONG

YOU
MATTER

Close your eyes.

Spin the book
around.

Put a finger
on the circle.

It speaks only
the truth.

(Magic!)

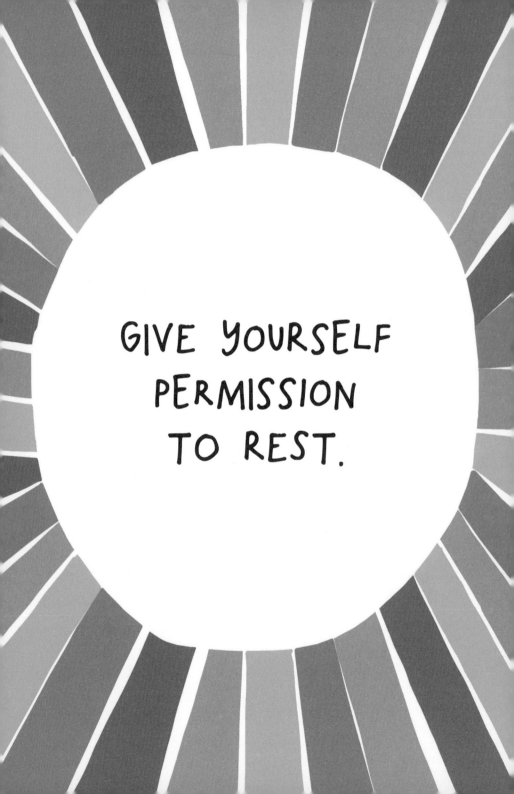

What are your favourite ways to rest and replenish?
What gets in the way of taking time out?

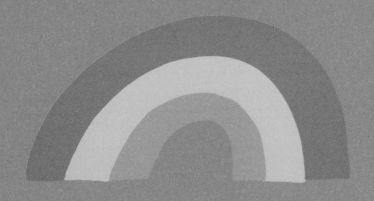

Set Social Media Boundaries

HEALTHY PHONE HABITS

Only follow accounts that uplift or inspire you

Set limits on your screen time

Delete apps for a social media cleanse

Turn off your notifications

Keep your phone out of your bedroom at night

My biggest ambition:

Qualities that will help me achieve my goal:

Help I need to ask for:

Skills I need to develop:

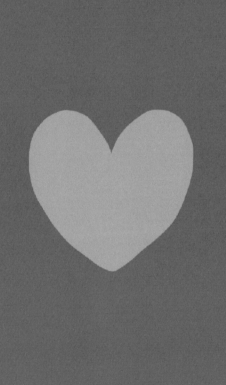

REMEMBER

IT'S OK TO TAKE UP SPACE

YOUR VOICE MATTERS

YOUR BODY IS MAGICAL

IT'S OK TO DEFY CONVENTION

YOU ARE WONDERFULLY UNIQUE

EMERGENCY SUNSHINE

TURN TO THIS PAGE OR
CUT OUT AND KEEP THIS
SUNSHINE TO BRIGHTEN
UP GLOOMY DAYS.

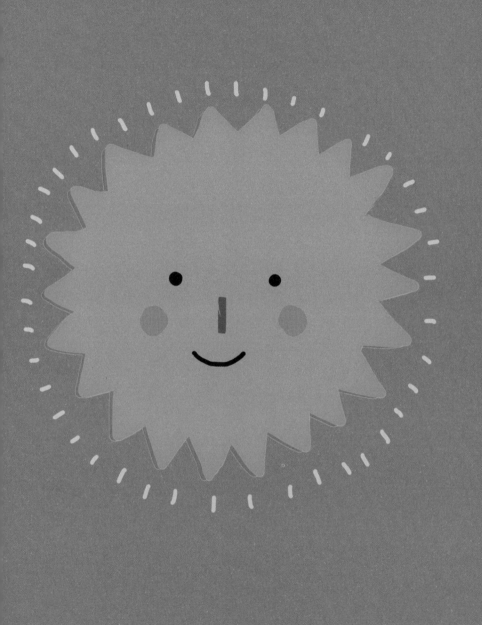

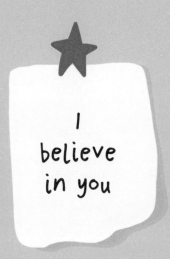

A little
note of encouragement

However you feel,

whatever you think,

You matter.

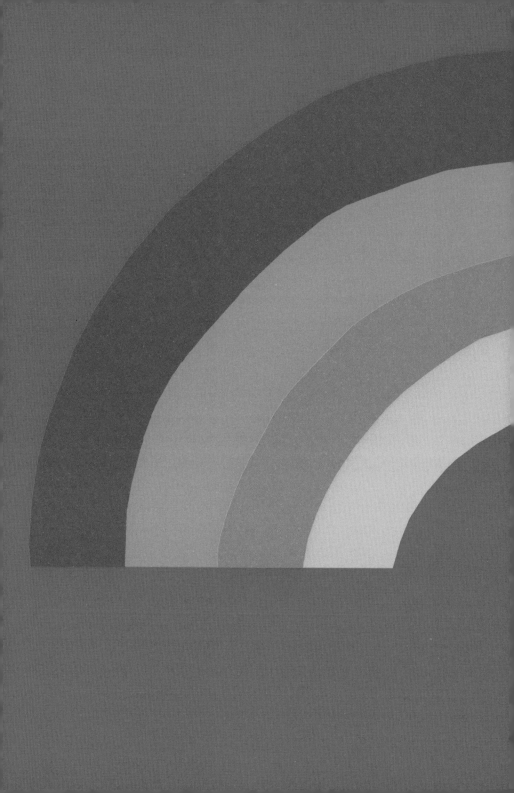

YOU ARE YOUR OWN
KIND OF WONDERFUL.

ONLINE KINDNESS CHALLENGE

Use social media for good and spread a
little bit of love and positivity each day
for a week.

You have the power to make a difference.

#PositivelyAwesomePrompts
#ThePositivelyAwesomeJournal

1) Leave an online review for your favourite local business

2) Share your favourite posts with tags and credit

3) Send your friends links to podcasts they might enjoy

4) Offer your support or skills to help someone in your online community

5) Send a happy DM. Let someone know you enjoy their work or content

6) Post a photo of the things you are most grateful for

7) Donate to or share the details of a charity or worthy cause

Other people's opinion of me

Likes and shares

The size of my body

I am more than

Grades and results

Past mistakes

My age

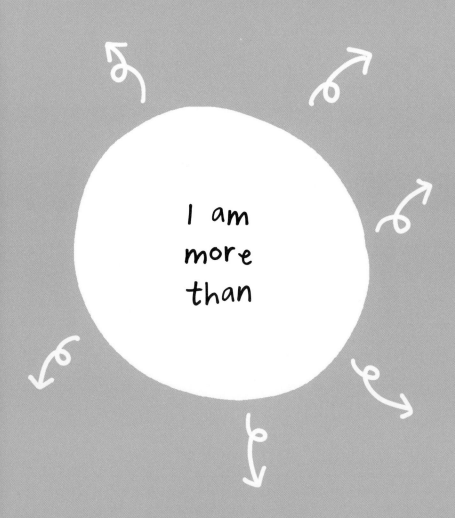

I am
more
than

We all like to feel valued and
know that we make a difference.

When have you felt most appreciated?

What words or actions made you feel
this way?

How do you demonstrate your appreciation for others?

If there are people who make you feel undervalued, how can you communicate this?

Remember: You are worthy, no matter how other people behave.

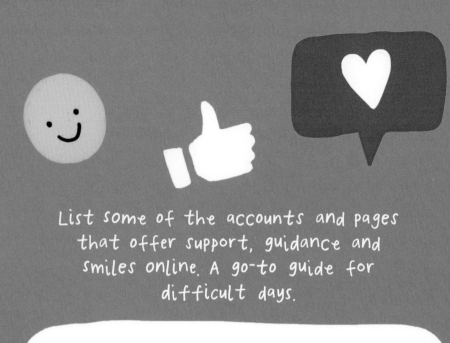

List some of the accounts and pages that offer support, guidance and smiles online. A go-to guide for difficult days.

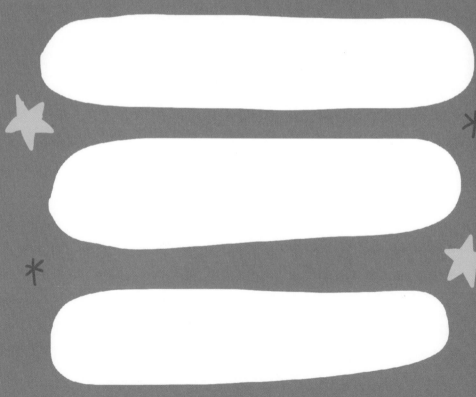

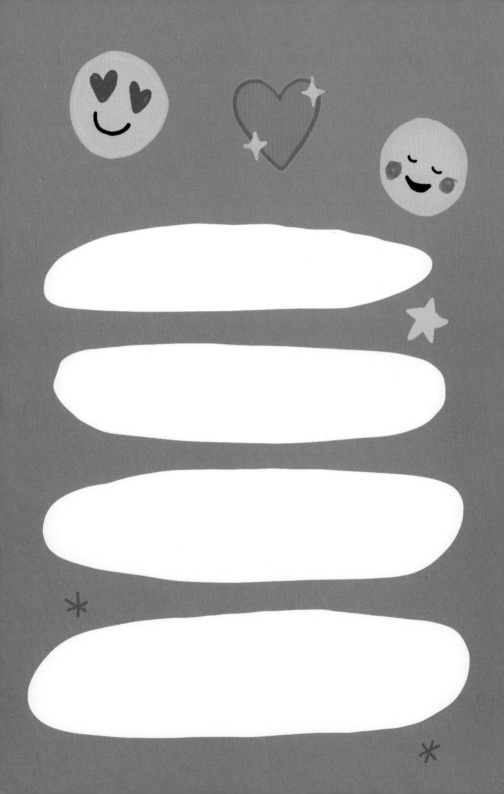

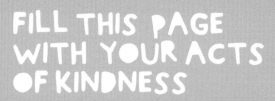

FILL THIS PAGE WITH YOUR ACTS OF KINDNESS

You make the
world brighter.

Create a city.
Make each building unique and individual.
There is beauty in difference.

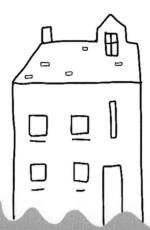

GROW CONFIDENT IN SAYING NO

What do you want to protect?

Who or what do you need to say no to?

What are some of the ways you can say no? Practise saying them out loud.

Don't compare yourself to others

Let yourself rest

Note the things you're proud of

SELF LOVE

Speak kindly to yourself

Let go of past mistakes

Say yes to things you love

You deserve your own love.
You deserve to treat yourself gently.
You deserve to speak to yourself
with respect and kindness.

We are all works in progress.

———

POSITIVELY AWESOME PROMPTS

Keep focused on your well-being by joining in with these prompts for social media posts.

Each one is inspired by a theme in this journal. Share a photo of a relevant page, create some artwork, write a blog post, share your sparkle and create a community online.

Choose them in any order and be as creative as you like!

Use the hashtag #PositivelyAwesomePrompts on your posts to join in.

We all experience ups and downs, let's continue to work through them.

#PositivelyAwesomePrompts

Self-care
Rainbow
Grow
Sparkle
Self-kindness
Enough
Nature
Gratitude
Progress
Space
Change
Dream
Rest
Self-love

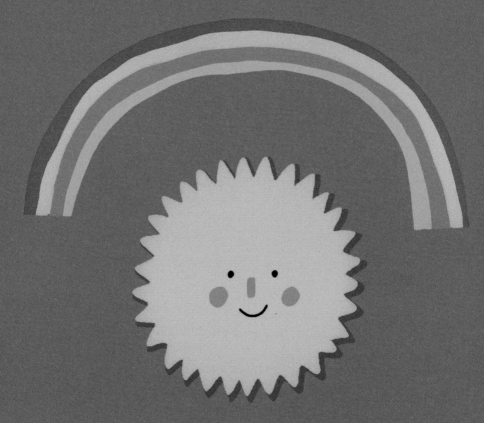

Find me online for more positive posts
and practical self-care prompts.
Stacie X

www.stacieswift.com
www.instagram.com/stacieswift

#ThePositivelyAwesomeJournal

#PositivelyAwesomePrompts

#StacieSelfCareChallenge